I0430239

Put Your Teenage Years Back to Your Penis

**Possess the Force of a Teenager
Via a No-Nonsense Way**

(Male Improvement Series)

————————

Creative Publishing

PUT YOUR TEENAGE YEARS BACK TO YOUR PENIS - Possess the Force of a Teenager via a No-Nonsense Way

Copyright © 2013 by Justin Perkins

All rights reserved. No part of this book may be reproduced or transmitted in any form or by any means without written permission from the author.

ISBN-13: 978-1484944387

ISBN-10: 1484944380

Printed in USA

There is a choice you have to make,
in everything you do.
So keep in the mind that in the end,
the choice you make, makes you.

-Anonymous

Dedication

This book is dedicated to my wife, Becky, who has given me all the support and understanding over the years.

This book is also dedicated to every man who wants more out of his life, even in the face of dealing with a personal problem at this level in his own hands.

Disclaimer

You should consult your physician or health care professional before making use of any suggestions included in this book to determine if you are the right candidate for such medications. This is particularly important if you (or your family) have a history of high blood pressure, heart disease, chest pain while exercising or have experienced chest pain in the past month when not engaged in physical activity, smoke, have high cholesterol or are overweight. Do not use the suggestions if your physician or health care provider advises against it. If you experience faintness, dizziness, pain or shortness of breath at any time please stop the program immediately.

Do not rely upon the information in this book as a substitute for professional medical advice, diagnosis, or treatment. If you have any concerns or questions about your health, you should always consult your physician or health care professional.

The use of any information provided in this book is solely at your own risk.

If you are in the United States and think you are having a medical or health emergency, call your health care professional or 911.

No one under the age of 21 should try anything detailed in this book.

Table of Contents

Preface

I suffered from ED (Erection Dysfunction) early on, in my 20s, the time most doctors were still blindly claiming that it was all in my head. I knew better what I was going through back then (1990s). Later it came the blue pill on the market with a stiff price tag (no pun intended, really). I did tons of research and found a similar route with a combination of 2 drugs (herbs) to induce erection at will during a 24-hour time frame – at a much reasonable cost.

I have taken it every day for more than 6 years now. It gets me ready like I had it in my teenage years. It was a "waste" for me when I was 15. I had all the force and power but didn't have a girlfriend to use it with every day. Now I have all the oomph back I can truly take advantage of and "bang" my wife on a daily basis. Life is incredible!

One of the purposes of this book is to broaden your horizon on this personal issue. Remember, there are other options you can take.

Introduction

The erection of a penis starts from getting stimulation - visual, psychological, and/or physical. When the brain receives the signals from stimulation, it then sends signals down the spinal cord. The nerve endings at the two spongy tubes in the penis (corpora cavernosa) then release the chemical compound nitric oxide into blood vessels of the corpora cavernosa and their surrounding tissues. The nitric oxide ignites the production of cyclic guanosine monosulphate (cGMP). cGMP relaxes the smooth muscles on the walls of the arteries that pump blood into the penis. More blood is then allowed to flow into the spongy tubes. On the other side, the walls of the veins carrying blood out of the penis contract, stopping the blood from flowing out of the penis. As the arteries are filled with blood, the penis expands and becomes longer, bigger and harder, producing an erection. There is an erection for the time the nerve endings in the spongy tubes receive signals from the brain. When the brain stops sending signals (due to the cease of stimulation or after ejaculation), an enzyme called phosphodiesterase (PDE5) is released, which causes the breakdown of cGMP. The walls of the veins carrying blood out of the penis relax, along with the smooth muscles in the artery walls to contract, reducing the amount of blood to flow into the penis. The penis is then back in the flaccid state.

Two contrasting groups of medicines created for relaxing and contracting arteries and veins have been in use by people managing their condition of high blood pressure and other problems.

This book takes you to have a closer look at these two drugs and their herbal equivalents.

The Bonus Chapters will give you inside details on how to increase your testosterone level safely, intelligently and stably, and how to improve Premature Ejaculation conditions, so that you can be well rounded inside and out.

Chapter One

So It Can Be Resolved

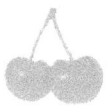

I intend to keep this book concise. I want to give you the much needed information – A key to the secret of an amazing sex life, in the fewest words possible.

Not only erection with spontaneity is preferred, heightened libido is much needed. Think back to your teenage years. The type of erection force and libido you had are godsend. You miss it, and now you want it back, no matter what age you are currently in, 20s, 30s, 40s, 50s, so on and so forth. So you will be surprised I will give you the key secret right up front, then work the way to other essential and significant supporting areas. Please heed, without these supporting factors fulfilled, things don't work the same, so be patient with me and read the entire book, from first page to the last.

My Own Story

I should be one of the most qualifying males to write this book. Why? I started suffering from ED in my mid-20s. Back then most doctors would want to take the easy way by telling you that it was all in your head. You ended up blaming yourself for the problem you had. "I had a lot of negative thoughts, so I couldn't get it up!" That was the 90s. Now in the second decade of the new millennium, we have better and more convincing figures. Psychological factors account for only about 10 to 20 percent of all erectile dysfunction cases; however, even these can sometimes be brought on as a secondary reaction to an underlying physical cause. With the latest medical findings, we now have a clearer understanding of what could contribute to an erection failure that haunts a man for a long time.

The Way It was Before the Year 1998

Before the market was introduced with drugs of PDE5 inhibitor in nature in 1998 (phosphodiesterase type 5 inhibitor), there were many medications for erectile dysfunction on the market that sort of helped some men but not others. One of the most known and used medicine back then was extracted from Yohimbe. While many men swore up and down that the herb, Yohimbe or the prescription drug Yohimbine helped them with their erection problem, many said that it didn't do anything for them at all.

What could be the factor that influenced the way Yohimbine worked in ED patients? Some had the penis up after taking it, and some failed to. Here you will find out how to make use of this herb/medicine in a way that it works every time. And I hear you. People have been saying how this herb could have undesirable side effects. Actually, the side effects can be avoided altogether.

Chapter Two

How Does It Work
&
Can We Mimic It?

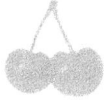

In 1998, a PDE5 inhibitor based medicine was introduced to the world. Suddenly all men around the world went crazy and tried to get their hands on this new drug. PDE5 is an enzyme that breaks down cGMP cycle, a regulator for the blood flow to the penis. In a nutshell, PDE5 is the show stopper. With PDE5, you don't have an erection.

So now it looks pretty straightforward that, by inhibiting or lowering the body's PDE5, a man gets an erection. Otherwise, a limp.

We now understand the basics of how a PDE5 inhibitor works. The next question is, is there a way we can mimic this inhibitor in an inexpensive way?

The Two Blockers that Work Wonders

Let's get a bit technical here. Contemporary research reveals that a coordinated interplay between the pathways of vasorelaxation and vasoconstriction shows a physiological mechanism that helps and maintains penile erection. Erection at the end is all about proper vasorelaxation and proper vasoconstriction. Luckily, coordinating both of these conditions is within our reach.

Medically, Yohimbine has a central alpha-2 blocking effect. This action can result in the increase of adrenaline and norepinephrine in the blood stream. In plain English, the main effects of adrenaline and norepinephrine on the body are to increase blood pressure and heart rate. This is what vasoconstriction does. On its own, what Yohimbine does not sound very well.

There is alpha-2 blocker, and there is also alpha-1 blocker, Prazosin. Prazosin is a type of vasodilator or vasorelaxant. Its job is to widen blood vessels. The result is the relaxation of smooth muscle cells within the vessel walls (an average penis smooth muscle percent is **between 40% and 50%),** especially in the large veins, large arteries, and smaller arterioles. This is what vasorelaxation does.

Here is the route as what happens in your penis after you take in alpha-1 and alpha-2 blockers at the same time.

The alpha-2 blocker, Yohimbine, increases the sympathetic outflow to the periphery which causes intense vasoconstriction. When the two alpha blockers are taken together, Yohimbine will override stimulation of peripheral alpha-1 blocker, Prazosin. Prazosin would hinder the action of Yohimbine to cause the blood pressure from rising. The combination has the unique properties of specifically enhancing cavernosal erectile function, preventing peripheral vasopressor alpha-1 and alpha-2 vascular receptors.

In lay person term, alpha-1 and alpha-2 blockers complement each other by canceling out the side effects of each other and at the end create a hard-on in a man.

Dosage

Each of us is different, controlled much by our genetic settings. Go slow and low with this combination of blockers in the beginning to create the spontaneous erection you crave for.

Yohimbine usually comes in at 6mg per tablet and Prazosin starts from 1mg per table. Go a quarter of each in the beginning, and check on your body's tolerance for them. Then increase by a quarter each time. Less can be more in this case.

Precautions

Diabetes: Yohimbine might interfere with insulin and other medications for diabetes and cause blood sugar dropping too low.

Schizophrenia: Yohimbine might worsen the condition of someone who suffers from schizophrenia.

Kidney Disease: Yohimbine might slow or stop the flow of urine.

Liver Disease: Preexisting liver disease might change the way the body processes Yohimbine.

Prostate-related Problems: Yohimbine might make the symptoms of Benign Prostatic Hyperplasia (BPH) worse.

Post-Traumatic Stress Disorder (PTSD): A report showing that PTSD patients suffered worse symptoms after using Yohimbine.

Chapter Three

Herbal Versions
Of
The Blockers

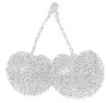

Both Yohimbine and Prazosin are prescription medicines. Many of you may not be able to get your hand on them. But then many of the medications in use are actually derived from plants or herbs. The blockers are no difference.

Herbal Yohimbine

It's well known that Yohimbine is extracted from Yohimbe (Pausinystalia Yohimbe), the plant. Yohimbe contains many other alkaloids; 55 of them have been found so far. Yohimbine is an alpha-2 only blocking agent which accounts for 1 to 20% of the total alkaloids.

Corynanthein is an alpha-1 only blocking agent found in Yohimbe. With alpha-1 blocker present in Yohimbe, the use of the herbal Prazosin should be reduced. Depending on the extract level, take about 760mg a day.

Herbal Prazosin

Extract of Opuntia ficus-indica flowers (NABIA extract) is an herbal form of alpha-1 only blocking agent, which can be used in place of Prazosin. Take about 1.5mg a day.

Precautions

Diabetes: Yohimbe might interfere with insulin and other medications for diabetes and cause blood sugar dropping too low.

Schizophrenia: Yohimbe might worsen the condition of someone who suffers from schizophrenia.

Kidney Disease: Yohimbe might slow or stop the flow of urine.

Liver Disease: Preexisting liver disease might change the way the body processes Yohimbe.

Prostate-related Problems: Yohimbe might make the symptoms of Benign Prostatic Hyperplasia (BPH) worse.

Post-Traumatic Stress Disorder (PTSD): A report showing that PTSD patients suffered worse symptoms after using Yohimbe.

Chapter Four

An Overlooked Way That Can Increase Testosterone

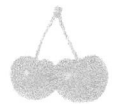

Erection is one thing; having adequate amount of testosterone running in the body is essential to maintain optimal level of libido, along with a few other masculine signs showing over the body. You must be amazed. Many people, males especially, do not pay much attention to this hormone-like vitamin, Vitamin D. Vitamin D, a fat-soluble vitamin exists in two major forms - vitamin D2 and vitamin D3. Vitamin D3 is most abundantly available as it is made by the skin when exposed to UVB radiations, as well as being available in certain dietary sources.

Increase the amount of vitamin D in your body to raise testosterone level, achieve a better body composition, and have better overall health.

Vitamin D3 synthesis can be triggered for production endogenously when ultraviolet rays from sunlight strike the skin. Some people have enough of it only because they get themselves exposed to the sun enough. In modern day belief, however, sun exposure is unhealthy - overexposure can cause skin cancer. To have ample vitamin D3 in the body, supplementing it seems to be the safest way. But hold on, why do we need to make sure we have enough vitamin D3 in the body?

At much closer look at the molecular level of vitamin D3's chemical structure, you will find a highly resemblance of the molecular structures of vitamin D3 and that of testosterone!

A study (published in **October 2011)** in the European Journal of Endocrinology tested vitamin D3 and hormone levels in 3051 men ranging from 40 to 79 years of age in Europe. Researchers found that men with vitamin D3 deficiency (below 50nmol/l or 20ng/ml) had significantly lower free testosterone. Adequate vitamin D3 to support optimal hormone

16

production was supplemented as there are vitamin D receptors in the hypothalamus and pituitary glands; both of them are involved in hormones production for metabolic and sexual health. And the major fact is men have vitamin D receptors in the testicles.

By supplementing this group with vitamin D3, the remarkable results came back. The total bioavailable testosterone levels increased as high as 25.2%.

Hundreds more studies have been made on this topic afterwards. They cover from muscle growth, fertility to erectile functions.

However, go low in the beginning. Try 400IU of Vitamin D3 along with about 20mg of magnesium. Work your way up to 5,000 IU vitamin D3 a day and up to 225mg magnesium a day.

I am not saying you should stay outdoors all the time from now on, or ditch your sunscreen on the beach. But deficiency in Vitamin D3 does lead to lowered testosterone levels.

No one can deny that supplementing vitamin D3 has to be the most overlooked, and the cheapest way to increase your testosterone levels.

What's Magnesium Got to Do with it

There could be side effects by taking vitamin D3? The answer is no, not really. There could be side effects, but they are the side effects of insufficient magnesium in the body.

To make vitamin D in the blood, your body must make use of magnesium. Males who are mildly to moderately magnesium deficient are commonplace. In such case, men who supplement with vitamin D3 and think that they are having vitamin D side effects are actually suffering from magnesium efficiency!

Here is a list of magnesium deficiency symptoms:

- Constipation (Vitamin D induced in insufficient magnesium environment)
- Jittery, hyperactivity, insomnia
- Anxiety (Vitamin D induced in insufficient magnesium environment)
- Palpitations
- Muscle cramps

Vitamin D Cofactors

When we supplement magnesium, depending on your diets, we could also tip off the balance of a few other elements in the body. There are a few things called vitamin D cofactors which the body needs to properly utilize all forms of vitamin D. If these cofactors are absent or on low in your body while supplementing vitamin D3, symptoms identical to vitamin D deficiency surface, namely fatigue, muscle aches, joint pain, depression, reduced immune system function and soft bones. It's mentioned above; the most interactive cofactor is magnesium. The other supporting cofactors are zinc, vitamin K2, and boron. All these are needed to achieve optimal results.

For zinc, you can take in up to 12mg a day. For vitamin K2, it is up to 800mcg. For boron, you need up to 3mg a day.

When there is a need, there is an answer. Many supplement/vitamin manufacturers produce vitamin D3 with addition of zinc, vitamin K2 and boron in one capsule. Browse online and you will easily a store that carries this type of vitamin D3 plus supplements.

Chapter Five

Stop Premature Ejaculation (PE)

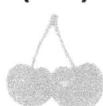

Up to this chapter, you may now be able to achieve an erection easily. But there lies another issue, you may say.

Premature ejaculation (PE) is more common than you realize. It can be embarrassing; the worst comes to it is that most often it is not considered significant enough to be treated by your doctor. There is no surprise that the actual number reported can be higher than this: About one third of sexually active men in the United States have this condition.

PE is stemmed from an ejaculation reflex in a man that is genetically pre-set at a lower, undesirable point.

On top of many autonomic and behavioral functions the neurotransmitter 5-HT also controls ejaculation. Through experiments, evidence shows that an enhanced synaptic availability of 5-HT in the central nervous system can assist in the control of ejaculation, depending on the enhancement level.

One of the prevalent methods many men who suffer from PE have tried: Lowering the penile hypersensitivity by applying topical anesthetic cream to the penis, resulting in partial anesthesia and the delay in ejaculation. The desensitizing creams create only numbness on the penis, which directly lowers the sensual enjoyment from love making. That's true. You would feel it as if wearing 10 condoms on your penis.

Adding enhanced synaptic availability of 5-HT in the central nervous system can be achieved by using an herbal extract, Hypericum perforatum. The name may look unfamiliar at first glance until I give

you the actual plant name, St John's Wort. It is the hyperforin extract of the plant that gives men this miraculous effect.

Only in the past few years have researchers discovered that hyperforin is the primary compound responsible for the mood-enhancing and delay ejaculation effect of St. John's Wort. You need the extract form of this herb to contain at least 3% of hyperforin for the satisfying effects. Remember though too much of hyperforin intake can cause serious delay in ejaculation and result in erectile dysfunction.

In a pilot study published in *The Internet Journal of Nutrition and Wellness*, 2007, we see that hyperforin extract of Hypericum perforatum lengthens the time of sexual intercourse before the man's ejaculation.

Precautions

Hyperforin can create side effects. It is important you notify your doctor before taking hyperforin if you are on other prescription medications such as mono amine oxidase inhibitors (MAOIs) or selective serotonin re-uptake inhibitors (SSRIs).

Chapter Six

A Few Things To
Pay Extra Attention To

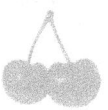

IFIS

Intraoperative Floppy Iris Syndrome (IFIS) has been observed in patients undergoing cataract surgery while being treated with alpha-1 blockers.

Dr. David F. Chang, clinical professor of ophthalmology at the University of California, San Francisco, School of Medicine, and researcher Dr. John Campbell tracked on 1,600 patients and found that conventional eye drops used in cataract surgery on patients with current or prior use of an alpha-blocker could not keep the pupil (the opening in the

iris) to stay completely open during cataract surgery.

According to Dr. Chang, there is no reason for those with cataracts to stop the medications before having surgery. Communicate with your eye surgeons the use of these drugs. This will allow the surgeons to take special precautions. "We can use different, longer-lasting dilation eye drops or micro-hooks to keep the pupil completely dilated during surgery," Chang said.

"You don't need to worry; you just need to inform your eye surgeon if you are currently taking, or have ever taken, Flomax or other alpha-blockers," said Dr. Chang.

The medical associations jointly issued a patient advisory regarding this on August 22, 2006.

Priapism

Priapism is the state of a penis having a sustainable erection that lasts over 4 hours and will not subside with ejaculation.

Priapism can lead to permanent impotence if untreated in a timely manner.

In very rare cases, alpha blockers are associated with priapism.

Priapism caused by using Prazosin has been reported in a few cases, and may be more likely in patients with renal insufficiency.

About the Author

Justin Perkins is a professional researcher who gets his hands on many levels of information in all possible areas, professions, fields and genres.

Let Justin know how you want the future editions of this book to have more and less on by sending your email to justingperkins@gmail.com

Upcoming Book

I am writing another book for the Male Improvement Series: **Go Multiple - Orgasmically**.

I don't need to say more, do I?

5-Star Review

If you think my book has helped you personally, please go to Amazon.com and give me a 5-Star review on the book. So that more people can find it and make use of it.

Thanks.

References and Further Reading

- **Regulation of pre-synaptic alpha adrenergic activity in the corpus cavernosum**
  - http://www.ncbi.nlm.nih.gov/pubmed/10845761
- **Method for treating impotence**
  - http://www.freepatentsonline.com/5567706.html
- **Dosage and inserter for treatment of erectile dysfunction**
  - http://www.google.com/patents/US5474535
- **Effect of vitamin D supplementation on testosterone levels in men**
  - http://www.ncbi.nlm.nih.gov/pubmed/21154195

- **Taking Too Much Magnesium**
  - http://www.livestrong.com/article/5034 89-taking-too-much-magnesium/#ixzz2RqX9X8mN
- **What are the Vitamin D Side Effects? You Might be Surprised**
  - http://www.easy-immune-health.com/Vitamin-D-Side-Effects.html#ixzz2RpWJyc9B

www.ingramcontent.com/pod-product-compliance
Lightning Source LLC
Chambersburg PA
CBHW070404290526
45790CB00004B/1634